GLAUCOMA

Clear Vision Ahead

Understanding

And

Managing Glaucoma

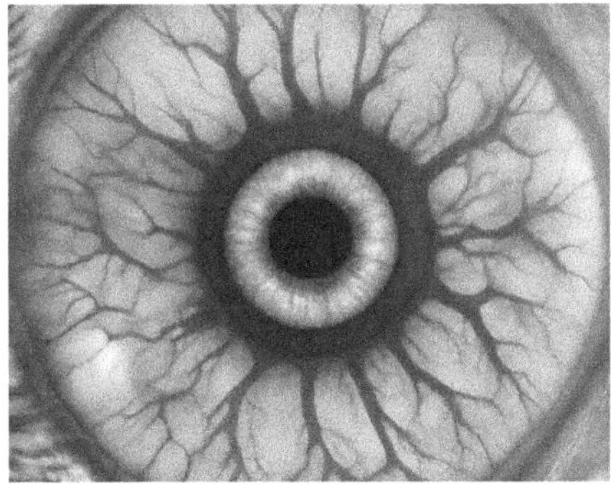

Dr. William G. Gomez

THANK YOU FOR CHOOSING US.

We Appreciate Your Kind Support And We Hope You Got Something Out Of It.

If You Enjoy This Book, It Will Be Great To Leave a **Review On Amazon** . It Means a Lot To Us.

Copyright © by Dr. William G. Gomez

2023.

Table of Contents

Have you ever pondered the preciousness of your sight, the intricate dance of light and perception that allows you to experience the vibrant world around you? Imagine a gradual dimming of that clarity, shadows encroaching on your once-clear vision. Now, consider the silent, often undetected, threat that is glaucoma – a condition that affects millions worldwide.

What if the key to preserving your eyesight lies in understanding the nuances of glaucoma? How can early detection make a pivotal difference? Join us on a journey through the corridors of ocular health as we unravel the mysteries of glaucoma, exploring its various forms, demystifying its causes, and discovering the crucial role of timely intervention.

In this exploration, we will delve into the mechanics of vision, uncover the treatment modalities available, and shed light on lifestyle adjustments that can complement medical approaches. As we embark on this enlightening journey, we aim not only to impart knowledge but also to empower you with the tools to navigate life with glaucoma, offering hope for a clearer tomorrow.

Whether you're personally affected by glaucoma, a caregiver, or someone eager to fortify their eye health, this guide is designed to be a beacon of understanding, providing insights, strategies, and a sense of assurance. Let's embark on this voyage together, where knowledge becomes a powerful ally against the shadows that threaten our vision.

Importance of Early Detection

1. Silent Development:

Glaucoma is known as the "silent thief of sight" because it grows slowly and without obvious symptoms in the early stages. Irreversible harm may have happened by the time symptoms appear. Early detection enables prompt management before serious vision loss occurs.

2. Vision Preservation:

The basic purpose of early detection is to keep eyesight intact. Glaucoma causes damage to the optic nerve, which transmits visual information to the brain. Early detection and treatment of the illness may stop or delay its growth, avoiding additional damage and preserving residual eyesight.

While glaucoma is treatable, treatment choices become increasingly restricted as the condition progresses. Medication, laser treatment, or surgical therapies may be beneficial in controlling intraocular pressure and managing the illness in the early stages. Late-stage glaucoma, on the other hand, may need more intrusive surgeries with a lower probability of regaining lost eyesight.

3. Enhancement of Quality of Life:

Maintaining strong eyesight improves a person's overall quality of life greatly. Individuals with early detection may continue to engage in everyday activities, drive, and enjoy hobbies without the significant limits that advanced glaucoma can impose.

4. Healthcare Cost Savings:

Glaucoma identification and control may result in more cost-effective healthcare. Regular eye examinations and early management are often less expensive than dealing with the effects of severe glaucoma, which may need extensive medical treatment, surgeries, and rehabilitation.

5. Personal and Economic Consequences:

Glaucoma-related vision loss may have serious emotional and economic effects.

Individuals may have difficulties in their work and personal life, affecting their independence and capacity to do everyday chores. Early identification aids in mitigating these effects.

6. Public Health Advantage:

Early identification and treatment of glaucoma contribute to a healthier and more productive society from the standpoint of public health. Regular eye tests and awareness efforts are critical in avoiding disease development on a larger scale.

CHAPTER 1

UNDERSTANDING GLAUCOMA

Glaucoma is a collection of eye disorders that cause damage to the optic nerve, the crucial connection between the eyes and the brain, and may result in vision loss or blindness. It is most usually linked with high intraocular pressure, although it may occur with normal or low pressure as well. Because the disorder is progressive and symptoms normally appear gradually, early identification and care are critical.

Glaucoma covers numerous varieties, each defined by specific characteristics, etiology, and development patterns. The two basic kinds are open-angle glaucoma and angle-closure glaucoma. Here's an overview of these key types:

- **Open-Angle Glaucoma:**

Description: This is the most prevalent kind of glaucoma, accounting for the majority of occurrences. It develops progressively over time as the drainage angle of the eye becomes less effective in enabling fluid (aqueous humor) to flow out.

Symptoms: Open-angle glaucoma is frequently asymptomatic in its early stages. Vision loss often happens gradually and may not be noticed until considerable damage has occurred.

Risk Factors: Advancing age, family history, African American or Hispanic ancestry, and certain medical problems such as diabetes.

Diagnosis and Treatment: Regular eye exams, including measuring intraocular pressure, examining the optic nerve, and visual field tests. Treatment comprises drugs (eye drops, oral), laser treatment, or surgical techniques to reduce intraocular pressure.

- **Angle-Closure Glaucoma**:

Description: This kind of glaucoma arises when the drainage angle of the eye gets blocked, creating an abrupt increase in intraocular pressure. It might be a medical emergency needing rapid treatment.

Symptoms: Sudden onset of acute eye discomfort, headache, blurred vision, nausea, and vomiting. This is in contrast to the sluggish growth of open-angle glaucoma.

Risk Factors: Hyperopia (farsightedness), age, and Asian or Inuit ancestry. It may also be connected with particular anatomical aspects of the eye.

Diagnosis and Treatment: Emergency medical intervention is required. Diagnosis requires monitoring intraocular pressure, examining the optic nerve, and imaging the drainage angle. Treatment may include drugs to lower intraocular pressure and laser or surgical techniques to clear the obstruction.

- **Normal-Tension Glaucoma:**

Description: In this kind, optic nerve injury and visual field loss occur despite intraocular pressure regularly measuring within the normal range.

Symptoms: Similar to open-angle glaucoma, it is generally asymptomatic until late stages.

Risk Factors: Similar to open-angle glaucoma, although the source of optic nerve injury in normal-tension glaucoma is not entirely known.

Diagnosis and Treatment: Regular eye exams, visual field testing, and optic nerve evaluation. Treatment focuses on reducing intraocular pressure with medicines or other measures.

- **Secondary Glaucoma:**

Description: Secondary glaucoma is a consequence of other eye disorders or systemic illnesses. It may arise as a consequence of accidents, inflammation, tumors, or drugs.

Symptoms: Vary depending on the underlying reason.

Risk circumstances: Presence of conditions or circumstances that lead to high intraocular pressure.

Diagnosis and Treatment: Addressing the root cause is key. Treatment may require drugs, surgery, or other procedures based on the unique circumstances.

Understanding the various kinds of glaucoma is critical for correct diagnosis and suitable therapy. Early identification and quick care are critical variables in protecting eyesight and avoiding additional impairment. Individuals at risk should receive frequent eye exams to monitor and manage their eye health properly.

THE MECHANICS OF VISION

- **How Glaucoma Affects the Eye**

Glaucoma affects the eye largely by destroying the optic nerve, a crucial component responsible for conveying visual information from the retina to the brain. The essential factors of how glaucoma affects the eye include:

1. Elevated Intraocular Pressure (IOP):

In many instances of glaucoma, there is an abnormal rise in intraocular pressure (IOP). This heightened pressure arises owing to a change in the equilibrium between the production and drainage of the aqueous humor, the fluid inside the eye. Elevated IOP is a primary risk factor for optic nerve injury in glaucoma.

2. Optic Nerve Compression:

Increased IOP may lead to compression of the optic nerve, especially at the point where the nerve fibers leave the eye. This compression limits blood flow to the optic nerve, decreasing its function and causing damage to the nerve fibers.

3. Optic Nerve Head Changes:

The optic nerve head, commonly known as the optic disc, undergoes structural alterations in glaucoma. These alterations commonly involve cupping, when the middle region of the optic disc gets larger. Cupping is a visual symptom of optic nerve injury and is often checked during eye exams.

4. Death of Retinal Ganglion Cells:

The optic nerve is formed of retinal ganglion cells that convey visual information to the brain. Increased intraocular pressure and other variables associated with glaucoma may lead to the death of these cells, causing irreparable damage to the optic nerve.

5. Visual Field Loss:

As the optic nerve suffers injury, visual field loss develops. Visual field loss in glaucoma frequently begins in the peripheral vision, leading to the progressive narrowing of the field of view. Individuals may not notice these alterations until the illness has advanced since center vision is initially retained.

6. Central and Peripheral Vision Affected:

While peripheral vision is often impacted early in glaucoma, as the illness worsens, it may also influence central vision. This might result in difficulty with activities that need acute, precise vision, such as reading or identifying faces.

7. Asymptomatic Nature:

One of the problems of glaucoma is its asymptomatic character in the early stages. Individuals may not feel discomfort or obvious symptoms, resulting in delayed discovery. Regular eye exams are critical for diagnosing glaucoma before irreparable vision loss occurs.

8. Different Types of Glaucoma:

The effect of glaucoma on the eye might vary based on the kind of glaucoma. For example, open-angle glaucoma, the most common kind, advances slowly and may not exhibit symptoms until later stages. In contrast, angle-closure glaucoma may lead to quick and severe symptoms owing to a fast rise in intraocular pressure.

a. Visual Field Loss

Visual field loss is a distinguishing symptom of glaucoma, a progressive eye illness that damages the optic nerve and may lead to permanent visual impairment. The visual field is the complete region that can be seen while the eyes are fixated on a central point. Here's an investigation of visual field loss in the context of glaucoma:

Peripheral Vision Affected:

In the early stages of glaucoma, the impairment often occurs in the peripheral or side vision. Individuals may not notice these modest alterations since central vision, which is critical for tasks like reading and recognizing faces, stays generally intact.

Gradual Progression:

Visual field loss due to glaucoma is frequently gradual and painless. This sluggish growth is one of the reasons why the illness is referred to as the "silent thief of sight." The progressive pattern of the loss highlights the significance of frequent eye exams for early diagnosis.

Visual Field Testing:

Visual field testing is an important diagnostic technique for measuring the level of visual field loss in persons with glaucoma. This test includes the display of lights or stimuli at different points within the visual field while the subject concentrates on a central point.

Scotomas and Blind Spots:

As glaucoma develops, patches of diminished sensitivity, known as scotomas, may appear in the visual field. These scotomas depict places where the individual's capacity to detect light or see things is hindered. Blind patches may also occur, resulting in problems in everyday tasks.

Tunnel Vision:

In the late stages of glaucoma, the visual field loss may lead to a condition known as tunnel vision. Tunnel vision confines the field of view to a tight cone, severely reducing peripheral vision. This substantially influences spatial awareness and the capacity to navigate the surroundings.

Challenges in Mobility and Activities:

Visual field loss may cause difficulty in actions such as driving, walking, and navigating congested environments.

Individuals may have trouble with identifying items or obstructions from the side, increasing the likelihood of accidents or crashes.

Quality of Life Impacts:

The effect of visual field reduction goes beyond physical activity. It may influence the general quality of life, leading to emotional and psychological issues. Restricted visual fields may lead to emotions of loneliness, anxiety, and a sense of dependency on others.

Importance of Early Detection:

Early identification of glaucoma via frequent eye exams is critical for avoiding or slowing down visual field loss. Timely intervention may assist in establishing ways to control the disease, conserving residual eyesight, and keeping a greater quality of life.

CHAPTER 2

TREATMENT OPTIONS

MEDICATIONS AND EYE DROPS

Several medicines and eye drops are regularly administered for the treatment of glaucoma. These drugs act by either decreasing the generation of intraocular fluid (aqueous humor) or enhancing its drainage, hence lowering intraocular pressure (IOP). It's vital to remember that the choice of medicine varies on the exact kind and severity of glaucoma. Here are some regularly used classes of glaucoma drugs and examples of individual eye drops:

1. Prostaglandin Analogs:
- These drugs improve the outflow of aqueous fluid, decreasing intraocular pressure. They are commonly

administered as first-line therapy owing to their effectiveness and once-daily dose.

Examples:

- Latanoprost (Xalatan)
- Bimatoprost (Lumigan)
- Travoprost (Travatan)

2. Beta-Blockers:

Beta-blockers lower intraocular pressure by reducing the formation of aqueous fluid. They are often used in conjunction with other drugs.

Examples:

- Timolol (Timoptic)
- Betaxolol (Betoptic)

3. Alpha Agonists:

Alpha agonists lower intraocular pressure by reducing aqueous humor production and boosting its outflow.

Examples:

- Apraclonidine (Iopidine)
- Brimonidine (Alphagan)

4. Carbonic Anhydrase Inhibitors:

These drugs lower intraocular pressure by reducing the formation of aqueous fluid. They may be administered as eye drops or taken orally.

Examples:

- Dorzolamide (Trusopt)
- Brinzolamide (Azopt)
- Acetazolamide (oral medicine)

5. Rho Kinase Inhibitors:

Rho kinase inhibitors enhance the outflow of aqueous fluid, helping to reduce intraocular pressure.

Example:

- **Netarsudil (Rhopressa)**

6. Combination Eye Drops:

Some drugs combine two or more types of glaucoma medications to simplify therapy and enhance compliance.

Examples:

- Dorzolamide-Timolol (Cosopt)
- Latanoprost-Timolol (Xalacom)

It's vital for patients with glaucoma to utilize their prescription eye drops as instructed by their ophthalmologist or healthcare practitioner. Adherence to the recommended regimen is critical for efficient treatment of intraocular pressure and avoidance of future optic nerve injury. Additionally, frequent follow-up sessions are important to evaluate the course of glaucoma and change the treatment regimen as needed.

Laser Therapy

Laser therapy is a widespread and successful treatment option for some kinds of glaucoma. It is typically applied to reduce intraocular pressure (IOP) and regulate the course of the disorder. Here's an overview of laser treatment in the context of glaucoma:

Types of Laser Therapy for Glaucoma:

❖ **Laser Trabeculoplasty:**
  - **Purpose:** Improving Aqueous Humor Drainage
  - How It Works: Laser radiation is given to the trabecular meshwork, the drainage angle of the eye, to improve the outflow of aqueous fluid. This helps to lower intraocular pressure.

Types:

- Argon Laser Trabeculoplasty (ALT) Selective Laser Trabeculoplasty (SLT)

❖ **Laser Iridotomy**:
  - Purpose: Treating Angle-Closure Glaucoma
  - How It Works: A tiny hole is produced in the peripheral iris using laser radiation. This incision enables the aqueous humor to flow more freely, alleviating pressure and minimizing rapid spikes in intraocular pressure.
  - Indications: Angle-closure glaucoma or diseases predisposing persons to angle closure.

❖ **Laser Cyclophotocoagulation:**
- Purpose: Reducing Aqueous Humor Production
- How It Works: Laser radiation is used to target and diminish the formation of

aqueous humor by treating the ciliary body, which creates the fluid.

- Indications: Usually reserved for more severe or resistant instances of glaucoma.

Key Considerations

Outpatient Procedure:

Laser treatment for glaucoma is normally conducted on an outpatient basis, and it frequently takes just a short period of time to complete.

Minimally Invasive:

Laser techniques are considered less invasive compared to standard glaucoma surgery. They are connected with fewer problems and a speedier recovery time.

Pain Management:

Discomfort during laser treatment is often mild. Some operations may need the use of topical or local anesthetic to ensure patient comfort.

Effectiveness and Duration:

The efficiency of laser treatment might differ among people. While some may have a considerable and persistent drop in intraocular pressure, others may need further therapies. The duration of the pressure-lowering action also varies.

Adjunct to Medications:

Laser treatment is commonly used as an adjuvant to glaucoma drugs. It may be advised when drugs alone are inadequate in managing intraocular pressure.

Follow-Up Monitoring:

Regular follow-up visits with an ophthalmologist are critical following laser therapy to evaluate the response to treatment, check any changes in intraocular pressure, and make modifications to the treatment plan if required.

Laser treatment plays a crucial part in the entire care of glaucoma. It is especially effective in circumstances when drugs alone may not give appropriate control or as a first therapy choice. The choice of laser treatment and the exact technique decided rely on the kind and severity of glaucoma, as well as the unique features of the patient's eyes.

SURGICAL INTERVENTIONS

Surgical procedures for glaucoma are explored when drugs and laser therapy are ineffective in lowering intraocular pressure (IOP) or when the disease is progressing despite conservative therapies. These surgical techniques try to develop new drainage channels for the aqueous humor or limit its production, thereby decreasing IOP. Here are some frequent surgical therapies for glaucoma:

Trabeculectomy:

- Purpose: To construct a new drainage route for the aqueous fluid by cutting a tiny hole in the sclera (the white area of the eye).

- How It Works: A tiny flap is formed in the eye's outer layer, enabling the aqueous humor to drain out of the eye and form a filtering bleb.
- Indications: Typically used for open-angle glaucoma when other therapies are not helpful.

Tube Shunt Surgery (Glaucoma Drainage Device):

- Purpose: To implant a tiny tube to transfer aqueous fluid from the eye to a reservoir (plate) under the conjunctiva.
- How It Works: The tube enables extra fluid to drain out of the eye, decreasing IOP.
- Indications: Used in situations of refractory glaucoma or when trabeculectomy is less likely to be effective.

Minimally intrusive Glaucoma Surgery (MIGS):

- Purpose: To lower intraocular pressure using less intrusive treatments with quicker recovery periods.

Examples:

- iStent: A small device inserted after cataract surgery to increase aqueous fluid outflow.
- Trabectome: Uses an electrocautery instrument to remove a part of the trabecular meshwork.
- Xen Gel Stent: A gelatin stent that forms a drainage route.
- Indications: MIGS operations are generally explored early in the therapy algorithm for mild to moderate glaucoma.

Cyclophotocoagulation:

- Purpose: To minimize the generation of aqueous humor by treating the ciliary body.
- How It Works: Laser radiation or freezing is administered to the ciliary body, limiting its capacity to generate fluid.
- Indications: Used in circumstances when alternative surgical procedures may not be acceptable or in refractory glaucoma.

Canaloplasty:

- Purpose: To boost the natural drainage system by opening Schlemm's canal.
- How It Works: A microcatheter is utilized to vasodilate and circumferentially open Schlemm's canal, enhancing aqueous humor outflow.
- Indications: Suitable for open-angle glaucoma, particularly those with mild to severe illness.

Ex-PRESS Shunt:

- Purpose: To produce a regulated drainage channel for aqueous fluid.
- How It Works: A small stainless steel device is implanted into the eye to assist aqueous fluid outflow.
- Indications: Considered in circumstances when traditional filtration surgery may have a greater risk of problems.

Considerations:

Postoperative Care:

- Surgical treatments need careful postoperative management and follow-up to monitor IOP, wound healing, and possible consequences.
- Risks and Benefits:
- The decision of surgical surgery relies on the kind and severity of glaucoma, as well as the patient's general condition. Surgeons analyze the risks

and advantages of each surgery to identify the most acceptable solution.

Individualized Approach:

The selection of a particular surgical surgery is generally tailored depending on the patient's unique circumstances, including the kind of glaucoma, past therapies, and overall eye health.

Surgical procedures for glaucoma serve a significant role in treating the condition and avoiding additional visual loss.

CHAPTER 3

LIFESTYLE AND GLAUCOMA

NUTRITION AND EYE HEALTH

Nutrition is essential for general health and has a substantial influence on eye health as well. Several nutrients and antioxidants are very good for eye health and lowering the incidence of eye-related disorders. Here are several important nutrients and their roles in eye health:

1. **Vitamin A:**
   - Role: Essential for preserving corneal health and encouraging healthy eyesight.
   - Sweet potatoes, liver, eggs, spinach, and kale are all excellent providers of this vitamin.

2. Zeaxanthin and Lutein:

- These antioxidants protect the eyes from high-energy light waves such as UV radiation.
- Leafy green foods (spinach, kale, collard greens), broccoli, peas, and eggs are good sources.

3. Fatty Acids Omega-3:

Supports retinal function and may aid in the prevention of age-related macular degeneration (AMD).

Walnuts, flaxseeds, chia seeds, and fatty fish (salmon, mackerel, and sardines) are excellent sources.

4. C vitamin:

- Function: An antioxidant that aids in the health of blood vessels in the eyes and may lower the likelihood of cataracts.
- Citrus fruits (oranges and grapefruits), strawberries, bell peppers, and tomatoes are also good sources.

5. Vitamin E:

- Protects cells from free radical damage and may help prevent age-related macular degeneration.
- Nuts, seeds, spinach, broccoli, and vegetable oils are all good sources.

6. **Zinc:**
- Important for retinal health and may aid in the prevention of age-related macular degeneration.
- Meat, dairy products, nuts, and legumes are all good sources.

7. Copper:
- Function: Collaborates with zinc to keep the optic nerve healthy.
- Seafood, nuts, seeds, and whole grains are good sources.

8. **Bioflavonoids:**
- Role: Collaborate with vitamin C to promote ocular blood vessel health.
- Citrus fruits, berries, onions, and tea are all sources.

9. **Antioxidants:**

Protect the eyes against oxidative stress and inflammation.

Colorful fruits and vegetables, such as berries, grapes, and leafy greens, are good sources.

Water:

Hydration is critical for maintaining fluid equilibrium in the eyes and avoiding dryness.

Water, herbal teas, and hydrating meals like fruits and vegetables are good sources.

Dietary Guidelines for Eye Health

- **Consume a Diverse Diet:**

Consume a variety of coloured fruits and vegetables to provide a wide range of nutrients and antioxidants.

- **Include Foods High in Omega-3s:**

For an excellent supply of omega-3 fatty acids, include fatty fish, flaxseeds, and walnuts in your diet.

- **Moderate Zinc Consumption**:

Consume zinc-rich foods in moderation, since excessive consumption may be harmful. Lean meats, dairy products, and lentils are all healthy sources.

- **Keep Hydrated:**

Drink plenty of water throughout the day to keep your body hydrated, especially your eyes.

- **Limit your intake of processed foods:**

Processed and high-sugar foods should be avoided since they may lead to inflammation.

- **Control Your Overall Health:**

Diabetes and hypertension, for example, may have an impact on eye health. Manage these illnesses with a healthy lifestyle and medical supervision.

- **Eye Exams regularly:**

While diet is important, frequent eye exams with a qualified eye care practitioner are critical for the early diagnosis and treatment of eye disorders.

A well-balanced and nutrient-dense diet, together with a healthy lifestyle, may considerably contribute to maintaining excellent eye health and lowering the risk of age-related eye diseases.

EXERCISE AND ITS IMPACT

Exercise has a key part in sustaining total health and well-being, and its influence extends to different facets of physical and mental fitness. Here's an investigation of the advantages of exercise across several dimensions:

Physical Health:

- **Cardiovascular Health**:

Regular exercise helps a healthy cardiovascular system by increasing heart and lung function. It helps minimize the risk of heart disease, high blood pressure, and stroke.

- Weight Management:

Physical exercise has a significant function in weight management by boosting calorie expenditure. Combining exercise with a healthy diet helps avoid obesity and associated health risks.

- Muscle Strength and Flexibility:

Resistance training and flexibility exercises promote muscular strength and joint flexibility, enhancing overall physical function and minimizing the risk of accidents.

- Bone Health:

Weight-bearing workouts, such as walking or strength training, enhance bone health by improving bone density and lowering the risk of osteoporosis.

- Improved Immune Function:

Regular, moderate-intensity exercise has been connected with a stronger immune system, lowering the risk of infections and boosting general resilience.

- Blood Sugar Regulation

Exercise helps manage blood sugar levels by improving insulin sensitivity. This is especially advantageous for persons with or at risk of type 2 diabetes.

Mental Health:

- **Mood Enhancement:**

Exercise boosts the production of endorphins, neurotransmitters that enhance feelings of pleasure and diminish symptoms of anxiety and despair.

- Stress Reduction:

Physical exercise functions as a natural stress reliever by lowering levels of stress chemicals like cortisol. It gives an outlet for pent-up energy and stress.

- Improved Sleep Quality:

Regular exercise is related to enhanced sleep quality and may help treat insomnia. It promotes a more peaceful and revitalising sleep.

- Cognitive Function:

Physical exercise has been connected with increased cognitive function, including greater memory, attention, and problem-solving abilities. It may also lessen the risk of age-related cognitive deterioration.

- Increased Energy Levels:

Regular exercise boosts overall energy levels and lowers symptoms of weariness. Engaging in physical exercise may be an excellent method for overcoming lethargy.

- Enhanced Self-Esteem:

Achieving exercise objectives and seeing gains in physical health lead to greater self-esteem and a good self-image.

- Social Well-Being: Social Connection:

Group activities, team sports, or fitness programs give chances for social contact, developing a feeling of community and support.

- Improved Relationships:

Engaging in physical activities with people may create social connections and enhance relationships. It gives common experiences and chances for interaction.

- Mental Resilience:

The discipline and drive established via regular exercise may contribute to mental resilience, helping people deal with life's problems.

Recommendations for Exercise:

Types of Exercise:

A well-rounded exercise regimen comprises a combination of aerobic activities (e.g., walking, running), strength training, flexibility exercises, and balancing exercises.

Frequency and Duration:

Aim for at least 150 minutes of moderate-intensity aerobic activity or 75 minutes of vigorous-intensity exercise each week, combined with muscle-strengthening exercises on two or more days a week.

Individualization:

Choose activities that match individual interests and health circumstances. Consult with healthcare providers, particularly for persons with pre-existing health difficulties.

Consistency:

Consistency is crucial. Regular, continuing exercise gives the most substantial advantages. Gradual growth and reasonable goal-setting lead to lasting habits.

CHAPTER 4

LIVING WITH GLAUCOMA

COPING STRATEGIES

Coping techniques are vital skills that people utilize to successfully manage and navigate through hard events, pressures, or life transitions. These practices contribute to emotional resilience, mental well-being, and general adaptive functioning. Here are numerous coping mechanisms that people might employ:

Emotional Coping Strategies: Mindfulness and Meditation:

Engaging in mindfulness techniques or meditation helps people remain present in the moment, decrease anxiety, and build a feeling of serenity.

Expressive Writing:

Journaling or expressive writing assists people in processing and releasing feelings. It may bring insights into moods and boost emotional well-being.

Deep Breathing Exercises:

Controlled deep breathing helps trigger the body's relaxation response, lowering tension and improving emotional stability.

Creative Outlets:

Pursuing creative hobbies, such as painting, music, or writing, gives a healthy outlet for emotions and self-expression.

Positive Affirmations:

Using positive affirmations may transform thinking patterns and promote a more hopeful outlook, improving resilience in the face of adversity.

Problem-Solving Coping Strategies:

Break Down Tasks:

Divide major activities into smaller, more achievable stages to make the effort feel less onerous.

Set Realistic Goals:

Establish attainable goals, then break them down into short-term and long-term targets. Celebrate minor wins along the road.

Seek Support:

Reach out to friends, family, or coworkers for advice, direction, or help. Sometimes, sharing difficulties with others might bring fresh views.

Time Management:

Organize tasks and prioritize them based on urgency and significance. Adequate time management can ease stress and enhance productivity.

Problem-Solving Techniques:

Utilize problem-solving approaches, such as brainstorming, to produce ideas and assess their practicality.

Social Coping Strategies:

Build a Support System:

Cultivate deep ties with friends and family to give emotional support during hard times.

Connect with Others:

Engage in social activities, join groups, or engage in group events to build a feeling of community and connection.

Share Feelings:

Openly discuss your opinions and emotions with trustworthy folks. Sharing the load may reduce stress.

Professional Support:

Seek professional help from therapists, counselors, or support groups when confronting complicated or chronic issues.

Physical Coping Strategies:

Regular Exercise:

Physical exercise produces endorphins, lowering stress and boosting general well-being. It also gives a chance for diversion.

Adequate Sleep:

Prioritize proper sleep hygiene to promote physical and mental well-being. Lack of sleep may worsen stress and weaken coping capacities.

Healthy Nutrition:

Maintain a balanced diet to promote general health. A proper diet adds to physical and mental resilience.

Relaxation Techniques:

Engage in activities that encourage relaxation, such as taking warm baths, doing yoga, or listening to peaceful music.

Cognitive Coping Strategies:

Cognitive Restructuring:

Challenge and reframe negative thinking patterns to build a more positive and productive mentality.

Mindfulness-Based Cognitive Therapy (MBCT):

Incorporate mindfulness with cognitive-behavioral tactics to boost self-awareness and encourage adaptive thinking.

Gratitude Practice:

Cultivate a practice of expressing thanks consistently. Focusing on good features might transform attitudes during stressful situations.

Humor and Laughter:

Find comedy in circumstances when appropriate. Laughter may function as a strong stress reliever.

Adaptive Coping Strategies: Acceptance:

Practice acceptance of conditions that cannot be altered. This may lessen emotional strain and assist problem-solving.

Flexibility:

Develop flexibility in thinking and adaptation to change. Being open to diverse outcomes develops resilience.

Self-Compassion:

Treat oneself with care and understanding. Avoid self-criticism, particularly during tough circumstances.

Learning and Growth Mindset:

Embrace adversities as chances for learning and personal improvement. Adopting a growth mindset builds resilience.

Remember that successful coping comprises a mix of these tactics, and their applicability may vary depending on individual preferences and the nature of the stressor. It's good to experiment with various strategies and discover what works best in particular scenarios.

ENHANCING QUALITY OF LIFE

1. Health and Wellness: Prioritizing physical health via regular exercise, balanced eating, and appropriate sleep creates the basis of a great quality of life. Physical well-being is strongly connected with mental and emotional fitness, producing a harmonious balance.

2. Mental and Emotional Well-Being: Cultivating healthy mental health is vital for a satisfying existence. Practices such as mindfulness, meditation, and stress management methods help with emotional resilience, self-awareness, and the capacity to face life's problems with a positive outlook.

3. Meaningful connections: Building and cultivating healthy, supportive connections with family, friends, and the community profoundly improves the quality of life. Meaningful friendships give emotional support, companionship, and a feeling of belonging.

4. Work-Life Balance: Striking a good balance between work and personal life is crucial. Avoiding burnout, establishing limits, and allocating time for leisure activities help to a more meaningful and sustainable existence.

5. Continuous Learning and Personal Growth: Engaging in continuous learning, following personal interests, and creating and attaining objectives lead to a feeling of purpose and personal satisfaction. Embracing difficulties and embracing chances for improvement are fundamental to a meaningful existence.

6. Financial Stability: Achieving a level of financial stability that meets basic needs and allows for discretionary spending on experiences and personal enjoyment positively impacts overall well-being. Financial stability alleviates stress and promotes the opportunity to follow one's interests.

7. Community Engagement: Actively engaging in community events, volunteering, or giving to social causes develops a feeling of connection and purpose beyond individual needs. Community participation provides a beneficial ripple effect, benefitting both individuals and the greater society.

8. Cultural and Recreational Activities: Exploring cultural experiences, engaging in hobbies, and enjoying recreational activities contribute to a rich and diversified quality of

life. These hobbies give possibilities for leisure, creativity, and self-expression.

9. Environmental Well-Being: A clean and sustainable environment adds to general health and well-being. Practices that encourage environmental stewardship, such as conservation and eco-friendly decisions, lead to a greater quality of life for current and future generations.

10. adaptation and Resilience: Developing adaptation and resilience in the face of life's uncertainties is vital for sustaining a high quality of life. The capacity to bounce back from obstacles and disappointments is an important part of psychological well-being.

PREVENTION AND REGULAR EYE CARE

Importance of Routine Eye Exams

1. Health and Wellness: Prioritizing physical health via regular exercise, balanced eating, and appropriate sleep creates the basis of a great quality of life. Physical well-being is strongly connected with mental and emotional fitness, producing a harmonious balance.

2. Mental and Emotional Well-Being: Cultivating healthy mental health is vital for a satisfying existence. Practices such as mindfulness, meditation, and stress management methods help with emotional resilience, self-awareness, and the capacity to face life's problems with a positive outlook.

3. Meaningful connections: Building and cultivating healthy, supportive connections with family, friends, and the community profoundly improves the quality of life. Meaningful friendships give emotional support, companionship, and a feeling of belonging.

4. Work-Life Balance: Striking a good balance between work and personal life is crucial. Avoiding burnout, establishing limits, and allocating time for leisure activities help to a more meaningful and sustainable existence.

5. Continuous Learning and Personal Growth: Engaging in continuous learning, following personal interests, and creating and attaining objectives lead to a feeling of purpose and personal satisfaction. Embracing difficulties and embracing chances for improvement are fundamental to a meaningful existence.

6. Financial Stability: Achieving a level of financial stability that meets basic needs and allows for discretionary spending on experiences and personal enjoyment positively impacts overall well-being. Financial stability alleviates stress and promotes the opportunity to follow one's interests.

7. Community Engagement: Actively engaging in community events, volunteering, or giving to social causes develops a feeling of connection and purpose beyond individual needs. Community participation provides a beneficial ripple effect, benefitting both individuals and the greater society.

8. Cultural and Recreational Activities: Exploring cultural experiences, engaging in hobbies, and enjoying recreational activities contribute to a rich and diversified quality of life. These hobbies give possibilities for leisure, creativity, and self-expression.

9. Environmental Well-Being: A clean and sustainable environment adds to general health and well-being. Practices that encourage environmental stewardship, such as conservation and eco-friendly decisions, lead to a greater quality of life for current and future generations.

11.adaptation and Resilience: Developing adaptation and resilience in the face of life's uncertainties is vital for sustaining a high quality of life. The capacity to bounce back from obstacles and disappointments is an important part of psychological well-being.

Tips for Eye Health Maintenance

1. **Regular Eye examinations:** Schedule complete eye examinations with an optometrist or ophthalmologist at least every two years. Regular check-ups are vital for early diagnosis of eye diseases.

2. **Protective Eyewear:** Wear safety glasses or goggles for activities that offer a risk of eye damage, such as sports, DIY projects, or certain work conditions.

3. **UV Protection**: Wear sunglasses that filter 100% of UVA and UVB rays to protect your eyes from sun-related damage.

Prolonged UV exposure may raise the risk of cataracts and other eye problems.

4. **Balanced Diet:** Consume a diet rich in eye-friendly nutrients, including vitamins A, C, and E, as well as omega-3 fatty acids. Incorporate lush greens, colorful fruits, seafood, and nuts into your meals.

5. **Stay Hydrated**: Maintain proper hydration to improve general eye comfort and avoid dry eye syndrome.

6. **Blink Regularly**: Practice the 20-20-20 rule while using digital devices: every 20 minutes, glance at someplace 20 feet away for at least 20 seconds. Blinking frequently helps avoid digital eye strain.

7. **Manage Screen Time:** Limit screen time and adjust screen brightness to prevent eye strain. Position displays at eye level to reduce discomfort.

8. **Quit Smoking:** Smoking is connected to an increased risk of age-related macular

degeneration (AMD) and cataracts. Quitting smoking improves greater eye health.

9. Eye-Friendly Workspaces: Ensure optimum lighting and ergonomics in your workstation to prevent eye strain. Position your computer screen at eye level and use suitable lighting to prevent glare.

CHAPTER 5

CASE STUDIES

SUCCESSFUL MANAGEMENT STORIES

Sarah, a vibrant and active individual in her mid-50s, first learned about her diagnosis of glaucoma during a routine eye examination. The news was unexpected, and she found herself navigating the complexities of a chronic eye condition that could potentially impact her vision.

Sarah's initial reaction was a mix of concern and uncertainty. The ophthalmologist explained the elevated intraocular pressure in her eyes and the importance of managing it to prevent further damage to the optic nerve. Sarah felt a sense of urgency to understand her condition and take proactive steps.

Adhering to the prescribed treatment plan, Sarah started using medicated eye drops to regulate intraocular pressure. The adjustment to incorporating eye drops into her daily routine came with challenges, but Sarah remained committed. Regular follow-up appointments with her eye care professional became a constant in her life, providing an opportunity to monitor the progression of the condition.

As the months passed, Sarah became adept at managing the practical aspects of living with glaucoma. She learned to recognize the importance of stress management in maintaining her overall well-being, as stress could potentially exacerbate intraocular pressure. Mindfulness practices and relaxation techniques became integral to her daily life.

One of the significant adjustments for Sarah was the need to adapt her lifestyle to minimize potential triggers for glaucoma progression. She paid extra attention to her diet, incorporating foods rich in nutrients beneficial for eye health. Regular exercise, while maintaining safety precautions, became a crucial aspect of her routine, promoting overall health.

Sarah's support network played a vital role in her journey. Her family and friends offered emotional support, understanding the challenges she faced. Attending local glaucoma support groups provided a sense of community and shared experiences, reinforcing the idea that she was not alone in this journey.

Despite the adjustments and occasional setbacks, Sarah's resilience shone through. She continued pursuing her passions, whether it was gardening, reading, or engaging in creative activities. Assistive technologies and tools designed for individuals with visual impairments became valuable allies in maintaining her independence.

Over time, Sarah's experiences with glaucoma became a narrative of strength, adaptability, and the importance of regular eye care. Through her journey, she realized the significance of staying informed, seeking support, and embracing a holistic approach to managing her condition. Sarah's story serves as an inspiration, illustrating that with proper care, a positive mindset, and a supportive community, one can navigate the challenges of glaucoma and lead a fulfilling life.

COMMON QUERIES ABOUT GLAUCOMA

1. What is Glaucoma?

Response: Glaucoma is a collection of eye disorders that damage the optic nerve, frequently owing to increasing intraocular pressure. It may lead to progressive visual loss and, if unchecked, may culminate in blindness.

2. How is Glaucoma Diagnosed?

Response: Diagnosis entails a full eye exam, including measuring intraocular pressure, examining the optic nerve, and visual field tests. Early discovery is crucial for an efficient cure.

3. What Causes Glaucoma?

Response: The specific reason is not usually evident, however, elevated intraocular pressure is a key risk factor. Other variables include age, family history, ethnicity, and certain medical problems.

4. Are There Different Types of Glaucoma?

Response: Yes, the two primary forms are open-angle glaucoma (more frequent) and angle-closure glaucoma. Other subtypes include normal-tension glaucoma and congenital glaucoma.

5. Is Glaucoma Hereditary?

Response: There is a hereditary tendency to glaucoma. Individuals with a family history of the disorder may have a greater risk, although it may also develop in individuals with no family history.

6. Can Glaucoma Be Prevented?

Response: While it cannot be totally avoided, early identification and care may delay its growth. Regular eye checkups, a healthy lifestyle, and minimizing risk factors contribute to prevention.

7. What are the Symptoms of Glaucoma?

Response: In the early stages, glaucoma frequently has no symptoms. As it advances, peripheral vision may be impaired. Regular eye check-ups are vital for early detection.

8. How is Glaucoma Treated?

Response: Treatment seeks to lower intraocular pressure. This might involve medicated eye drops, oral drugs, laser therapy, or surgery, depending on the severity and type of glaucoma.

9. Can Vision Loss from Glaucoma Be Restored?

Response: Unfortunately, eyesight loss from glaucoma is permanent. Early identification and care are critical to avoid additional impairment and maintain residual eyesight.

10. How Often Should I Have an Eye Exam for Glaucoma?

Response: The frequency varies on numerous variables, including age, family history, and general eye health. Generally, persons should undergo frequent eye checkups every 1 to 2 years.

11. Can Glaucoma Be Managed Without Medication?

Response: In certain circumstances, lifestyle adjustments such as regular exercise, a balanced diet, and avoiding tobacco might complement medical therapy. However, checking with an eye care specialist is crucial.

12. Is Glaucoma More Common in Older Adults?

Response: Yes, the risk of glaucoma rises with age. However, it may afflict persons of any age, including youngsters.

13. Are There Any Risk Factors for Glaucoma?

Response: Yes, various risk factors include age (especially over 60), family history, African or Hispanic origin, high intraocular pressure, thin corneas, and certain medical problems like as diabetes and cardiovascular disorders.

14. Can Glaucoma Develop Suddenly?

Response: While glaucoma normally grows slowly and frequently without symptoms, acute angle-closure glaucoma may occur unexpectedly and cause fast vision loss. This is considered a medical emergency needing quick care.

15. How Does Glaucoma Affect Vision?

Response: Glaucoma frequently affects peripheral vision initially, progressing to tunnel vision in severe stages. Central vision may stay clear until later phases. Regular eye examinations are critical for early identification before obvious vision loss occurs.

16. Can Lifestyle Changes Help Manage Glaucoma?

Response: Yes, some lifestyle modifications may complement medical therapies. Managing stress, having a balanced diet rich in antioxidants, frequent exercise, and avoiding tobacco may help general eye health.

17. Is Glaucoma Linked to Other Health Conditions?

Response: There are correlations between glaucoma and other health disorders, like as hypertension and diabetes. Managing these disorders is crucial for general health and may favorably improve glaucoma treatment.

18. Can Glaucoma Be Treated Surgically?

Response: Yes, surgical procedures may be needed for specific types of glaucoma.

Procedures such as trabeculectomy, laser trabeculoplasty, or implantation of drainage devices attempt to lower intraocular pressure.

19. Is It Safe to Use Contact Lenses with Glaucoma?

Response: Individuals with glaucoma may typically wear contact lenses safely. However, it's vital to discuss this with an eye care specialist who can give advice depending on the individual kind and severity of glaucoma.

20. Can Glaucoma Medications Have Side Effects?

Response: Yes, like all drugs, those used to treat glaucoma may have negative effects. Common adverse effects include redness, inflammation, or changes in the color of the eyes. Regular follow-ups with an eye care specialist assist in monitoring and treating any adverse effects.

21. Can Glaucoma Lead to Blindness?

Response: If left untreated, glaucoma may lead to permanent visual loss and, in extreme circumstances, blindness. However, with early discovery and adequate therapy, the course of the illness may be delayed or prevented, averting major visual damage.

22. Is Glaucoma Painful?

Response: In most situations, glaucoma is not unpleasant. The absence of obvious symptoms in the early stages is one reason frequent eye examinations are vital for early diagnosis.

23. Can Glaucoma Be Present in Both Eyes?

Response: Yes, glaucoma may affect one or both eyes. It typically advances at different rates in each eye, underscoring the significance of regular eye examinations for monitoring both eyes.

24. Are There Support Groups for Individuals with Glaucoma?

Response: Yes, there are local and online support groups where persons with glaucoma may share experiences, acquire insights, and get emotional support. Organizations such as the Glaucoma Research Foundation typically give tools and information on support networks.

Conclusion: Embracing Vision and Hope

As we conclude this journey through the intricacies of glaucoma, we hope that this book has served as a valuable resource, offering insights into the complexities of the condition and empowering you with the knowledge to navigate its challenges.

Glaucoma, often referred to as the "silent thief of sight," demands our attention, understanding, and proactive engagement. From the fundamentals of eye anatomy to the intricacies of diagnosis, treatment, and lifestyle management, we have explored the various facets of this eye condition. Throughout these pages, we have emphasized the importance of early detection, regular eye care, and the role each individual plays in preserving their vision.

Remember, knowledge is a powerful tool, and with it comes the ability to make informed decisions about your eye health.

Regular eye examinations, open communication with healthcare professionals, and adherence to treatment plans are key components of managing glaucoma effectively. As we've delved into the stories of those living with glaucoma, we've witnessed resilience, adaptability, and the unwavering spirit of individuals determined to maintain their visual well-being.

In the pursuit of better eye health, it is essential to stay informed, seek support from healthcare professionals, and actively engage in a holistic approach to wellness. Your journey with glaucoma is unique, and by embracing the knowledge within these pages, we hope you find the tools to face the challenges with courage and optimism.

Let this not be the end but rather a new beginning—a beginning marked by understanding, empowerment, and a commitment to the precious gift of sight. As we look toward the future, filled with advancements in research and treatment options, may your path be illuminated with the light of knowledge, and may your vision remain clear and bright.

Wishing you a future filled with vision, hope, and a life well seen.

www.ingramcontent.com/pod-product-compliance
Lightning Source LLC
Chambersburg PA
CBHW061007260726
48661CB00005B/2091